looking back at ...

CLASSIC

•CORONATION ST.•

1960-1990

Published by Cognitive Books Limited,
115 New Road, Croxley Green WD3 3EN. United Kingdom
Published by Cognitive Books, 2024

This book has primarily been developed and published for those living with dementia and their loved ones. This is not intended to be an official history of *Coronation Street*. However, every attempt has been made to research the topic thoroughly and any inaccuracies are unintentional.

We are committed to working with print partners who prioritise environmental and social responsibility. Printed and bound in Latvia by PNB Print.

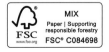

looking back at ...

CLASSIC

·CORONATION ST.·

1960-1990

Written by Matt Singleton
Illustrations by Simon Reid

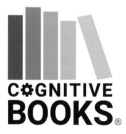

COGNITIVE
BOOKS®

Download the free audio version of this book at cognitivebooks.co.uk/download or by scanning the QR code.

If you're the supporter (e.g. a carer or a loved one) of the person reading this book, you can enjoy it too! There are some useful hints and tips for you on pages 76 and 77 of this Cognitive Book to make sure everyone gets the most out of it.

Become a Cognitive Bookworm at cognitivebooks.co.uk

This book has been created in collaboration with Alzheimer's Society. 5% of the publisher's proceeds from the sale of this Cognitive Book will be paid to the charity. The aim of Cognitive Books is to increase this contribution over time. ITV Studios Ltd has worked with Cognitive Books to help create this unique book for their loyal viewers over the years.

You can find lots of useful information about Alzheimer's Society and their work at alzheimers.org.uk and more about ITV at itv.com

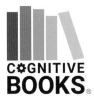

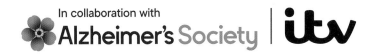

For Colleen, a *Corrie* fan and loving wife to my dad.
Thank you for all you do to support him.

With special thanks to Dad (Brian) as always, Graeme, Richard, Sarah, Jenna, Kirsty and the team at Alzheimer's Society, AJ, Christina, Dominic, Helen, Sian and the team at ITV, Simon, Daisy, Liz, Rebecca, Kirsty, Nicky, Nicola, Chris, Ros, Clarissa, Megan, Alex, Pippa, Sam and the CBL team, my colleagues at Swiss Re and – as ever – Claire, William, Ben and (for her occasional and welcome companionship while I work) Smidge The Cat.

Matt Singleton, 2024

In loving memory
Jeanette 'Nettie' Singleton (née Andrews)
1939-1986

CONTENTS

Foreword — 7

The story of Classic *Coronation Street*, 1960-1990 — 9

Exercises — 39

   Just for fun – it's quiz time — 40

   Some more quiz questions — 45

   Did we know? — 48

   Let's chat — 52

Exploring Weatherfield further — 55

   Coronation Street map — 56

   Coronation Street through the decades — 58

   Quick facts — 64

   Go further into the world of *Coronation Street* — 68

   Quiz answers — 69

All about me — 74

Supporters' guide — 76

FOREWORD

Dear Reader,

Because it touches so many of our lives, both of ITV's soap operas have run important stories with dementia at their heart: most notably *Coronation Street* with Mike Baldwin and *Emmerdale* with Ashley Thomas.

We've always tried to infuse these stories with lighter moments of humour, of personal connection and of deep affection, showing the dementia journey for what it is: sometimes painful but sometimes, also, life affirming. The one thing dementia does do is remind us how important those around us are: family, friends, community and carers – how much they mean to us and how much we mean to them. And that is also the central message of a soap like *Coronation Street*.

All of this underlines the importance of *Corrie* being part of this initiative and we hope this book will help stir fond memories of a soap, which many millions have enjoyed and shared over the years: with their family and friends, both on screen and off.

John Whiston
Managing Director, Continuing Drama, ITV Studios

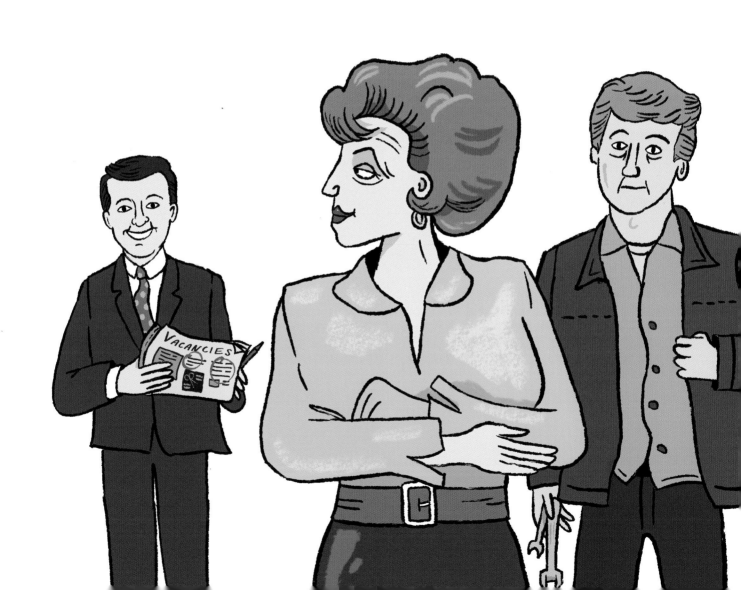

THE STORY OF CLASSIC CORONATION STREET, 1960-1990

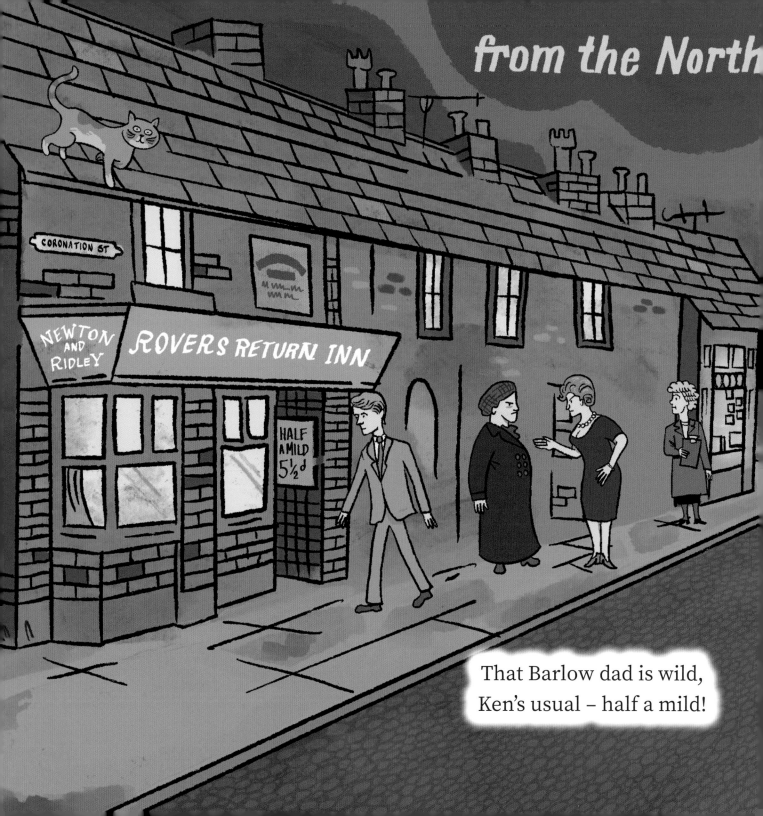

The first episode:
INTRODUCTION TO THE STREET, 9TH DECEMBER 1960

Brass wails out from our telly sets, there's folk with 'Up North' vocals,
Through the streets of Weatherfield, it's time to meet the locals.
They're buying on the never-never, they're quite like you and me,
Florrie at the Corner Shop; the Barlows at Number Three.
Ken aspires to the middle class, it's driving his dad wild!
Young Barlow's soon off down the pub, for his usual (half a mild).
There's the Tanner–Sharples feud, about them we'd soon learn,
To our TVs we're now glued and, like The Rovers, we'd Return.

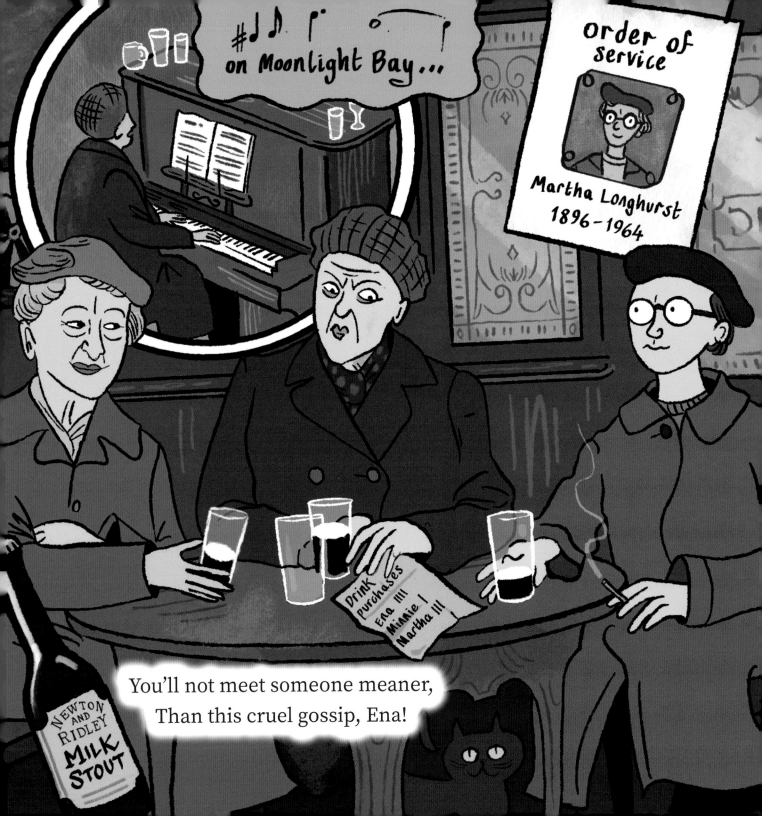

The Rovers Return regulars:
ENA SHARPLES, MINNIE CALDWELL, MARTHA LONGHURST

A hair-netted cruel gossip, you'll not meet someone meaner,
There are no words in edgeways, if talking back to Ena.
Flanked by Minnie and Martha, the pensioned working classes,
It's always dear old Minnie's round, with Martha there in glasses.
In the confines of the snug, the three will talk about,
Other people's business, over bottled milky stout.
That is until one sad old day, when Martha's in her chair,
A singalong, 'On Moonlight Bay', she slumps and dies right there!

Watching *Coronation Street*,
The greatest of the soaps,
From The Kabin to The Rovers,
A world of fears and hopes.

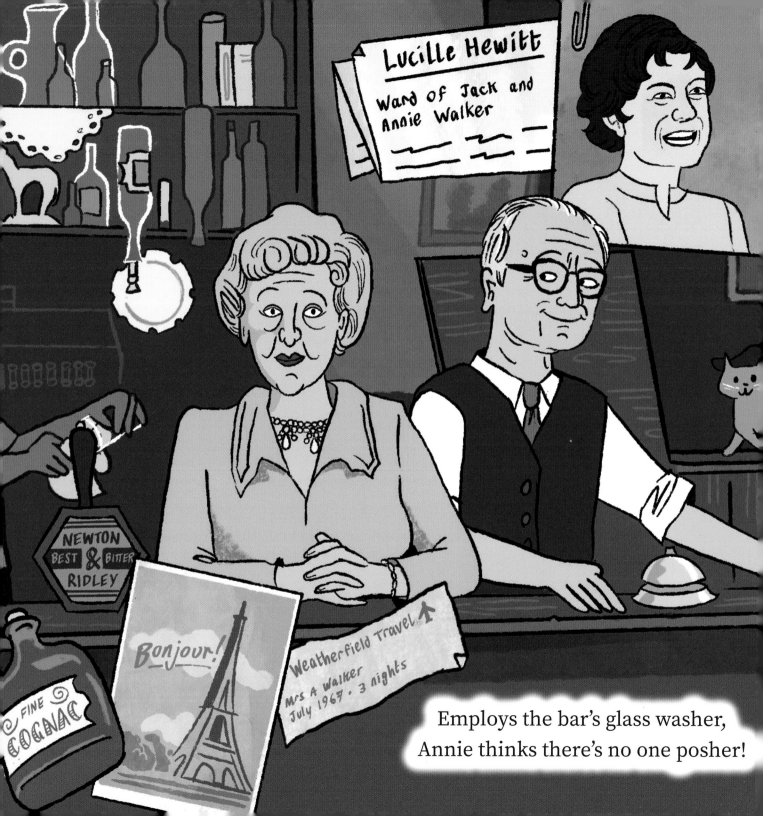

Employs the bar's glass washer,
Annie thinks there's no one posher!

Legendary landlady one:
ANNIE WALKER

Rules the roost, employs so many: the bar staff, the glass washer,
Wants to dress like she's the Queen, she thinks she's even posher.
Looks up to the gentry, looks right down on the meek,
Thinks that she's Parisienne – was in France less than a week!
But Annie and Jack are gentle folk, though it seems they'd break through steel,
They help in the community, they take care of Lucille.
After her husband's heart attack, poor Annie's left alone,
She struggles on without her Jack, then lives with daughter, Joan.

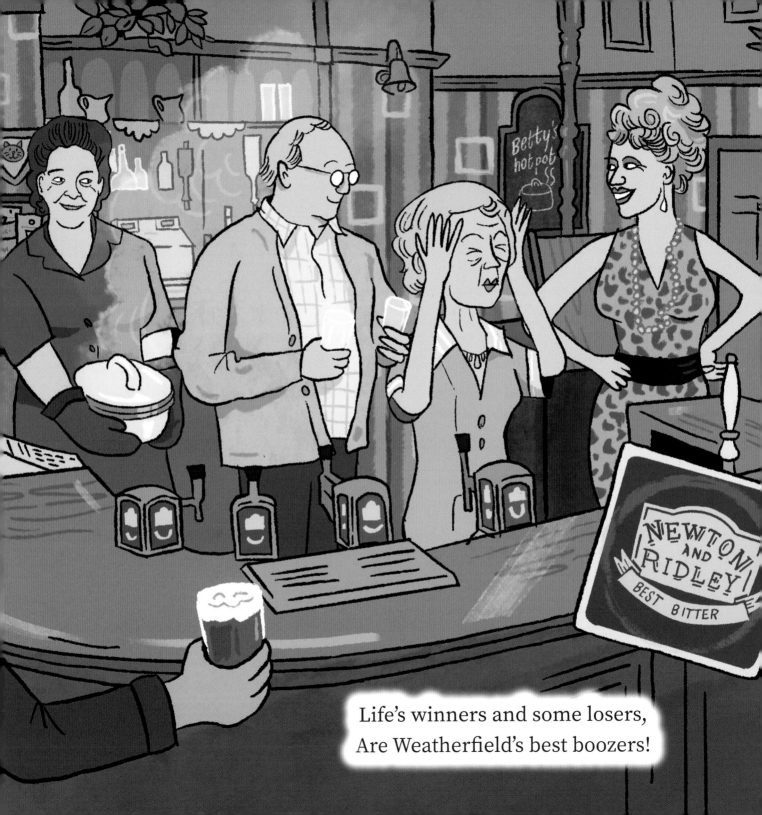

Life's winners and some losers,
Are Weatherfield's best boozers!

THE CLASSIC ROVERS BAR STAFF LINE-UP

The Rovers hosts our characters, life's winners and some losers,
There's always something going on among Weatherfield's best boozers.
Bet and Betty's banter, makes Annie Walker frantic,
She winces at another joke about a neighbour's bedroom antic!
Poor old Fred, the potman, he does fancy his chances,
But Bet will tease and laugh it off, ignoring his advances.
Newton and Ridley's finest ale, their drinks can pack a punch,
A local pub that cannot fail, with Betty's hotpot lunch.

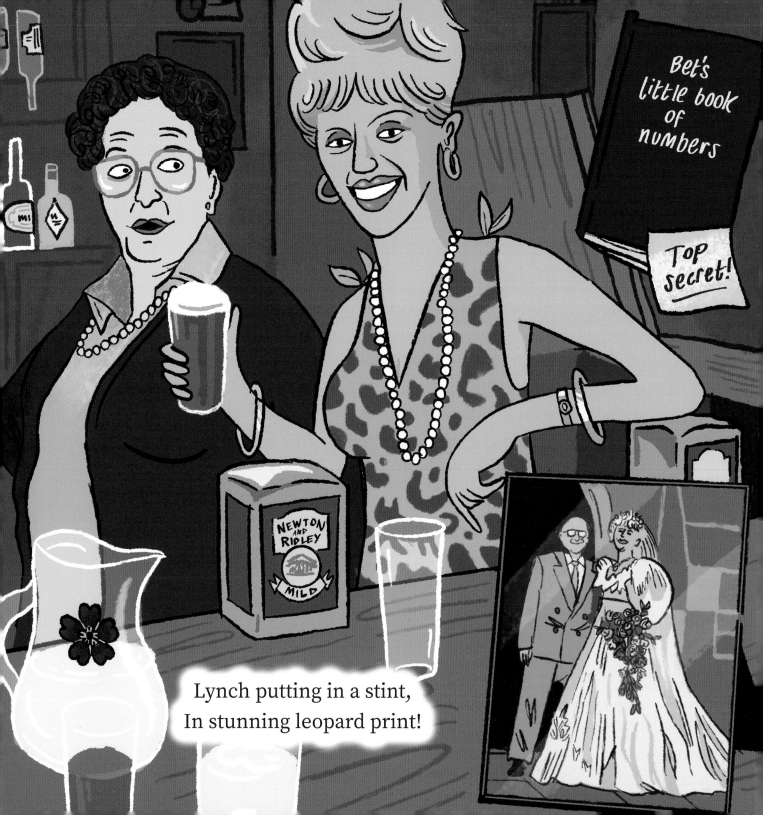

Lynch putting in a stint,
In stunning leopard print!

Legendary landlady two:
BET LYNCH

All those years behind the bar, Lynch putting in a stint,
The former local Beauty Queen, in stunning leopard print.
Vulnerable but tough outside, from the school of life's hard knocks,
She shrugs it off, and she'll admit, she's been around the blocks.
Along comes Alec Gilroy, he knows her reputation,
They're brave enough to tie the knot, to the joy of every patron!
We want the best for our dear Bet, a thousand four-leaf clovers,
The finest, picturesque sunset, the ruler of The Rovers.

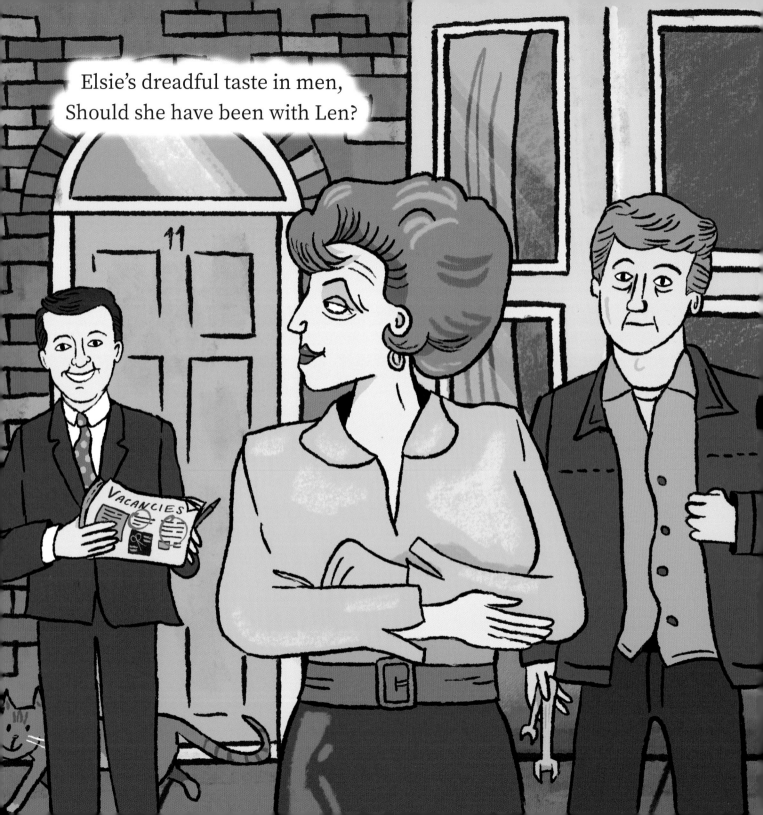

The tough lass:
ELSIE TANNER

All those accusations fly, she's taken for a ride,
A grandmother at thirty-eight, some man's bit on the side.
But Elsie Tanner's fiery, she deals with every menace,
Warpaint on, with flame-red hair, and a hapless son called Dennis.
Ena and Annie turn their noses at her dreadful taste in men,
The American does not work out, should she have been with Len?
It all goes wrong right up until, she can finally afford,
To confess her love to suitor, Bill, they leave to live abroad.

Watching *Coronation Street*,
The greatest of the soaps,
Weatherfield just seems so real,
A world of fears and hopes.

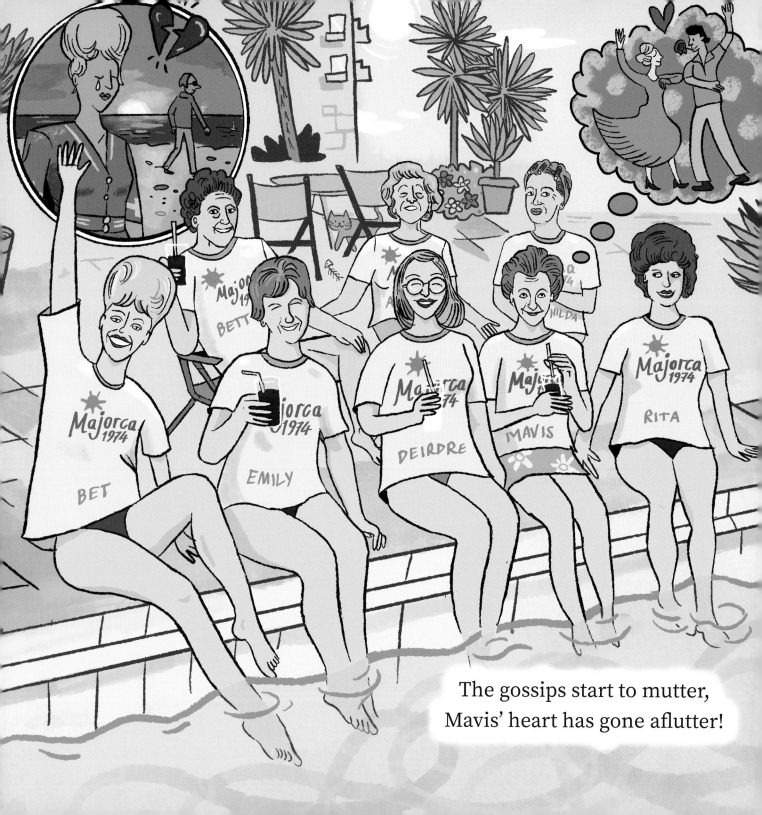

The gossips start to mutter,
Mavis' heart has gone aflutter!

The ladies of *Coronation Street*:
1974's TRIP TO MAJORCA

A holiday competition, Bet's betting group has won,
How else would you get this motley crew heading for the sun?
There's Rita, Mavis, Bet and Hilda, of course there's Annie Walker,
Deirdre, Betty and Emily, raise the heat up in Majorca!
Pedro falls for Mavis, the gossips start to mutter,
A stolen kiss at flamenco night! Her heart has gone aflutter.
Bet bags herself a fancy man, their talk is rather steamy,
Soon it goes right down the pan, it doesn't end all dreamy.

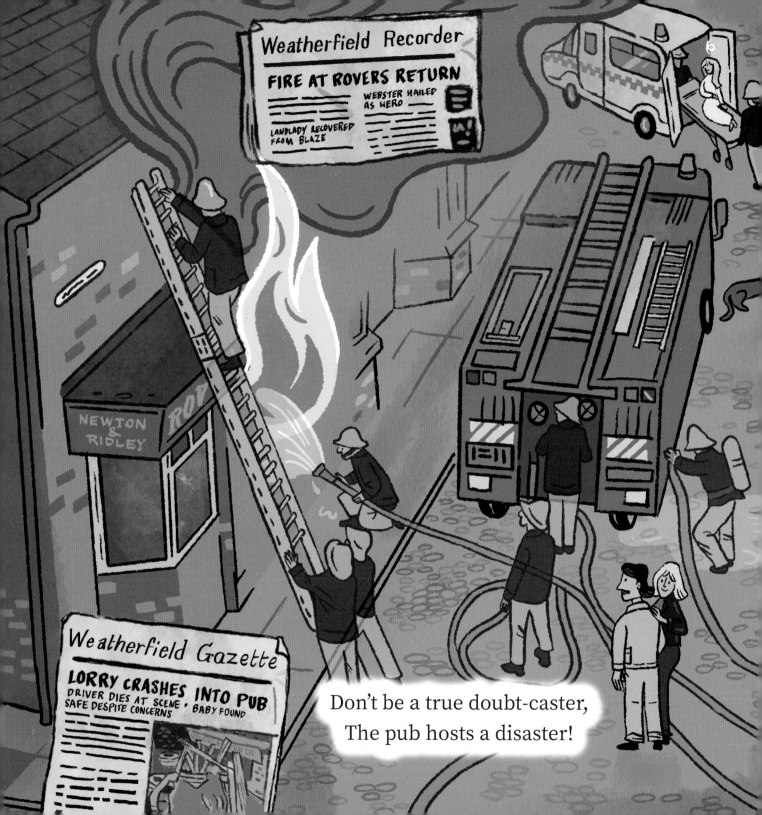

DISASTERS ON THE STREET

Don't say The Street is blessed with luck, all of you doubt-casters,
We couldn't know one single pub would host all these disasters!
A lorry crashes into it, causing death of driver,
Deirdre breathes a sigh of relief, baby Tracy's a survivor.
There's a fire at The Rovers and Bet Lynch is trapped inside,
Kevin Webster rescues her, much to Sally's pride!
It's caused by faulty wiring, Jack's blamed for the bad news,
All those sparks are firing, and Bet then blows her fuse!

Watching *Coronation Street*,
The greatest of the soaps,
Twice a week, we'd tune in,
To a world of fears and hopes.

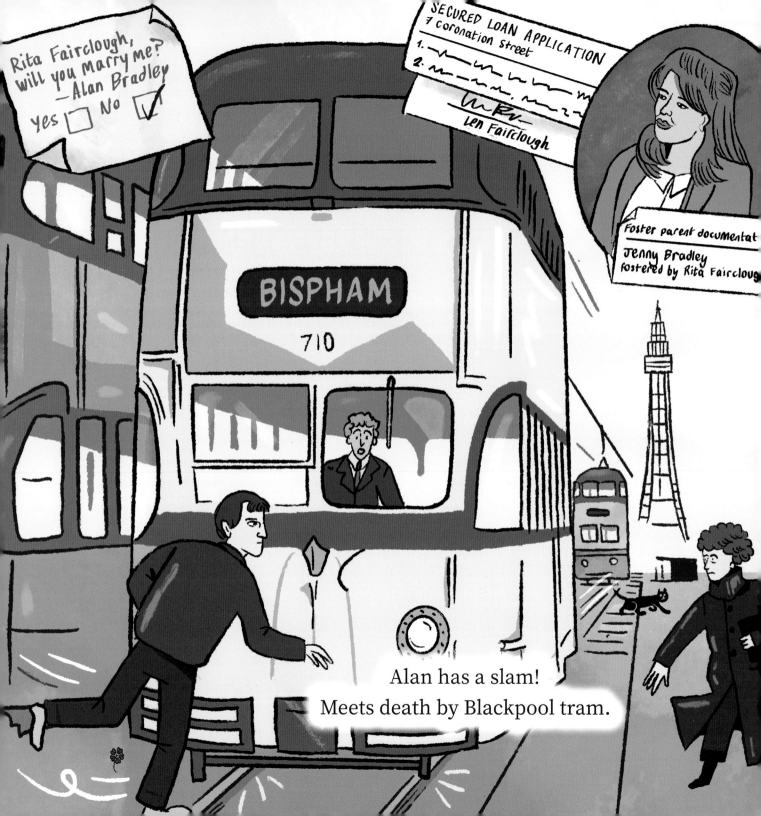

The disastrous relationship of ...
ALAN BRADLEY
AND RITA FAIRCLOUGH

Mrs Fairclough has a heart, Jenny's fostered by our Rita,

She falls for Jenny's father, a liar and a cheater.

She refuses Alan's proposal: no registrar, no church,

He poses as her husband, Len, who's long since left his perch.

He defrauds her of a ton of cash, a sinister gameplay,

A court case finds him guilty; he walks free on the same day!

His harassment of poor Rita, ends up with a slam!

That nasty woman beater, meets death by Blackpool tram.

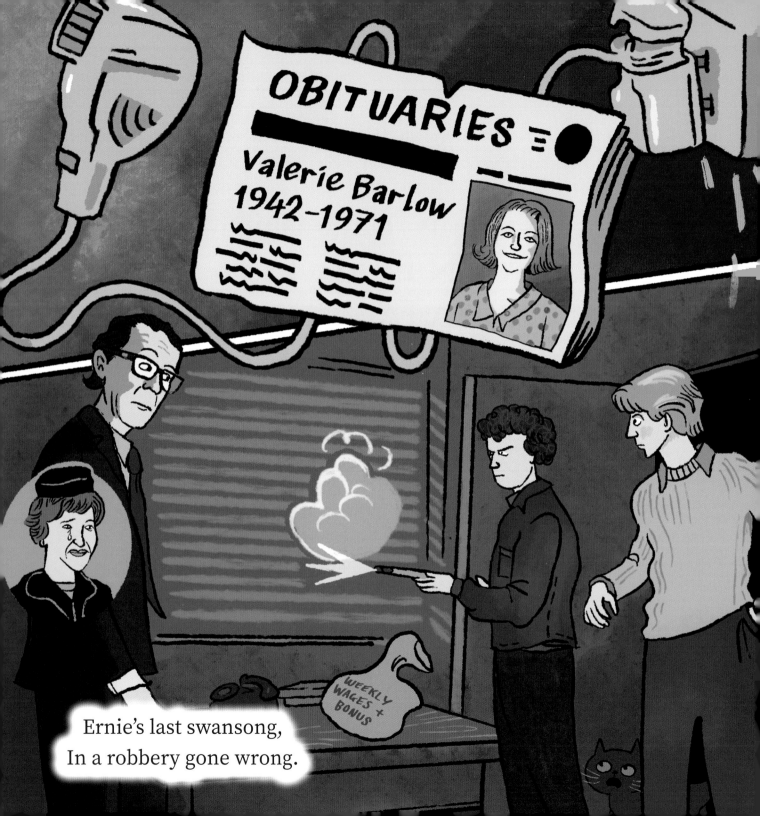

DEATHS ON THE STREET

You can't escape the reaper, whether butcher or a baker,
On The Street there's no nice way to go and meet your maker!
Valerie and Ken Barlow have become an institution,
That is until it ends for her: horrific electrocution!
The aftermath is rather brutal, their maisonette's on fire,
Who'd have thought that this mayhem could be caused by one hairdryer?
Emily Bishop's sadly widowed, for Ernie his swansong,
A shotgun, a lamenting ode, in a robbery gone wrong.

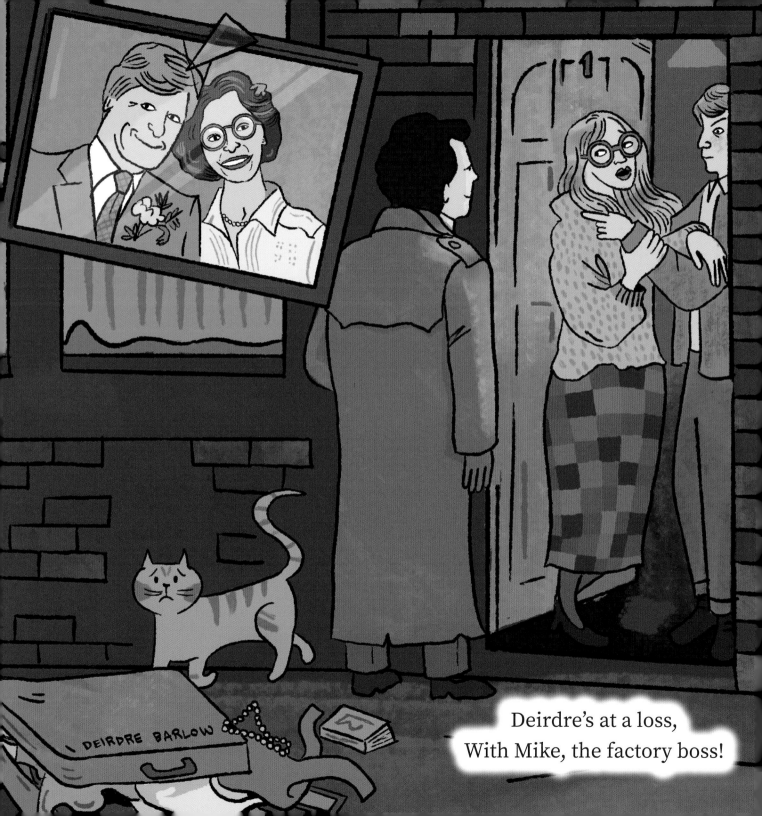

Deirdre's at a loss,
With Mike, the factory boss!

The couple's scandal:
DEIRDRE AND MIKE'S AFFAIR

Ken is self-absorbed, in his own life and career,
The needs of his wife, Deirdre, go in and out each ear.
The loneliness, the drudgery, she seems all at a loss,
But then along comes Baldwin, the local factory boss.
Her affair she soon confesses, she can't maintain her silence,
And sure enough, when Mike comes round, it nearly turns to violence!
She raises the white flag, she hesitates and then,
Though told to pack her bag, our Deirdre chooses Ken.

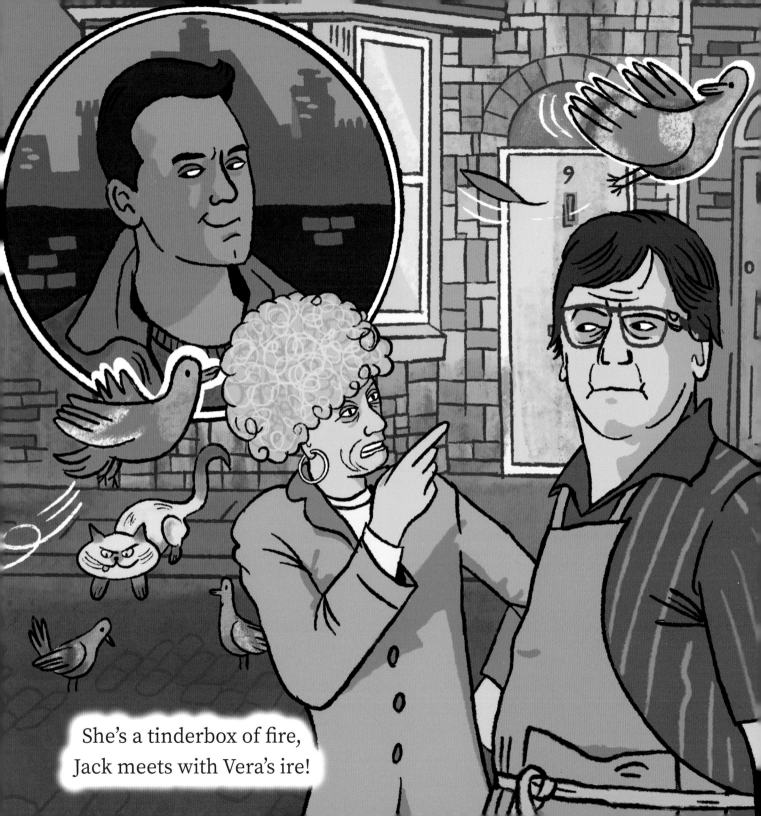

She's a tinderbox of fire,
Jack meets with Vera's ire!

Classic couple one:
VERA AND JACK

Jack thinks that he's a ladies' man, the pub is his religion,
But there's nothing that he fancies more than a racing pigeon!
He meets his match in Vera, a tinderbox of fire,
She catches him out so frequently and unleashes her ire.
Vera's pride at Number Nine, the tasteless things she's adding,
The residents upon The Street detest the Duckworths' cladding!
But their love for one another, upon their cake that cherry,
The frustration of a mother, with a roguish son like Terry.

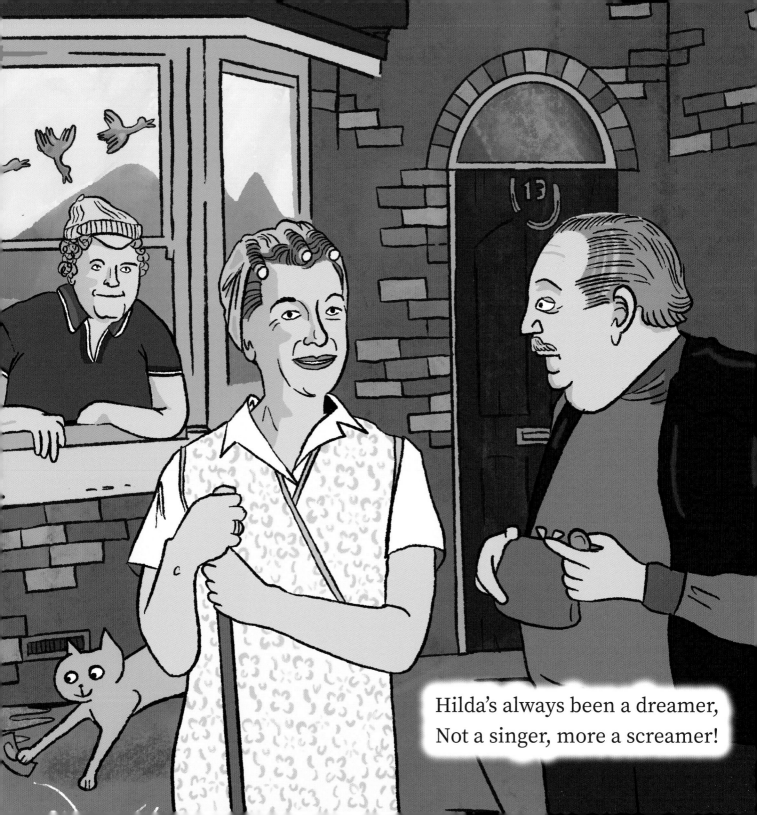

Classic couple two:
HILDA AND STAN

Hilda wants life's luxuries, but she's always been a dreamer,
Scrubbing on her hands and knees, no singer, more a screamer!
With rollers, headscarf, housecoat too, her Stan's a pro work-dodger,
Scraping pennies, ducks on wall, with Eddie Yeats as lodger.
Stan's glass back does not prevent him scamming his dear wife,
Anything to sup a pint, and to have an easy life.
But Stan and Hilda really care, they're caught when they do fall,
It turns out those with nowt to spare, are the richest of them all.

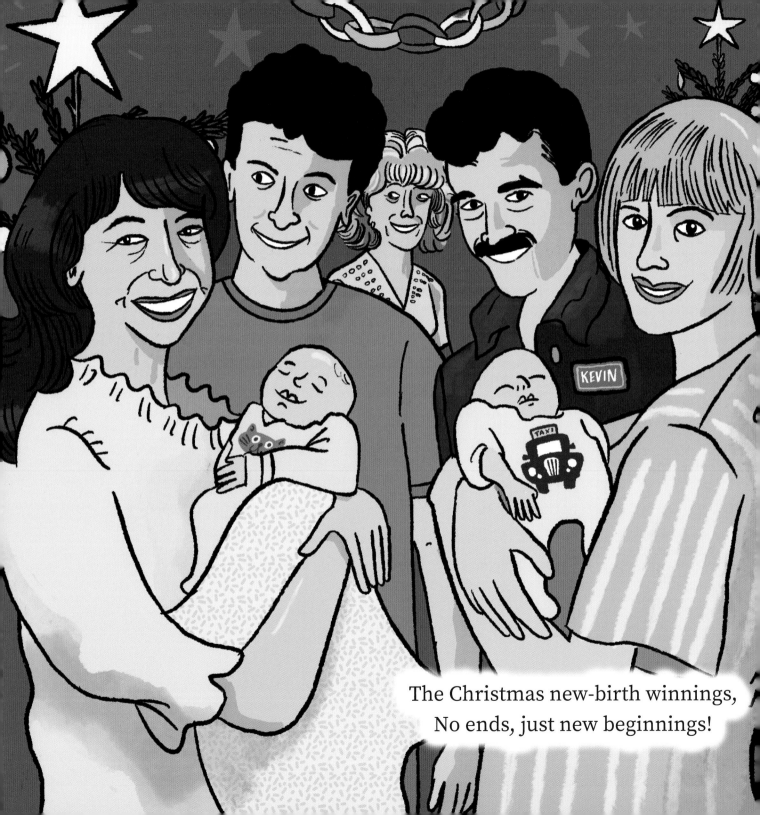

The Christmas new-birth winnings,
No ends, just new beginnings!

BIRTHS ON THE STREET, CHRISTMAS 1990

The stork can sometimes pay a visit to *Coronation Street*,
Bearing gifts of brand-new life (pitter-patter, tiny feet).
One Christmas we meet two young faces, one in Don Brennan's cab,
Rosie Webster joins the clan, it's Kev and Sally's bab.
Nicky and Sarah Lou's Christmas gift, is David, their kid brother,
Gail and Martin, mum and dad, and Audrey proud grandmother.
All this joy that new life sends, the Christmas new-birth winnings,
And just like *Corrie*, it never ends, there's only new beginnings.

Watching *Coronation Street*,
The greatest of the soaps,
A reflection of life and our true selves,
A world of fears and hopes.

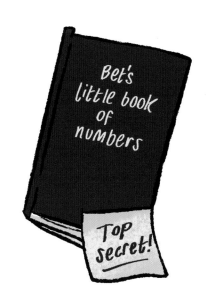

EXERCISES

Just for fun – it's quiz time!

These questions are from the story and all the answers can be found in the book!
You get one mark for each with a total of fourteen points to get.
The answers are on page 69-70.

The first episode: Introduction to The Street, 9th December 1960 (page 11):

What is the name of the fictional town in which *Coronation Street* is set?

a. Weatherfield
b. St Florrie's
c. Barlowsville

The Rovers Return regulars: Ena Sharples, Minnie Caldwell, Martha Longhurst (page 13):

Which of the Ena, Minnie and Martha trio wears glasses and dies in her seat at The Rovers Return?

a. Ena
b. Minnie
c. Martha

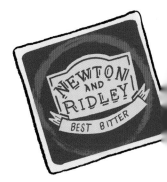

Legendary landlady one: Annie Walker (page 15):

Who is put into the care of Annie and Jack Walker as their ward after her dad, Harry Hewitt, and stepmum, Concepta, move to Ireland?

a. Lucille
b. Jemima
c. Joanna

The classic Rovers bar staff line-up (page 17):

What in-demand lunch dish is Betty Turpin renowned for at The Rovers Return?

a. Mulligatawny soup
b. Chicken curry
c. Lancashire hotpot

Legendary landlady two: Bet Lynch (page 19):

Who does Bet marry when they tie the knot in 1987?

a. Don Brennan
b. Alec Gilroy
c. Jack Duckworth

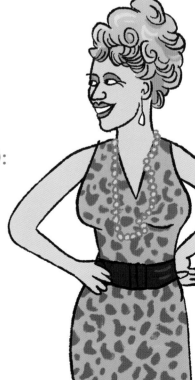

The tough lass: Elsie Tanner (page 21):

Is this statement true or false? Elsie Tanner became a grandmother at the age of thirty-eight.

  a. True

  b. False

The ladies of *Coronation Street*: 1974's trip to Majorca (page 23):

Which seemingly innocent character has a romantic kiss with Pedro at a flamenco night on the ladies' trip to Majorca?

  a. Rita

  b. Deirdre

  c. Mavis

Disasters on The Street (page 25):

What is the name of Deirdre's baby daughter, who is feared missing when a lorry crashes into The Rovers Return?

  a. Tracy

  b. Stacy

  c. Maisy

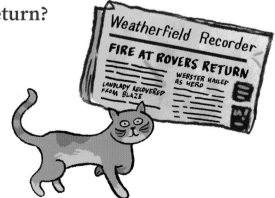

THE DISASTROUS RELATIONSHIP OF ALAN BRADLEY AND RITA FAIRCLOUGH (PAGE 27):

In which seaside town does Alan meet his end, after being hit by a tram?

    a. Blackpool

    b. Camber Sands

    c. Weston-super-Mare

DEATHS ON THE STREET (PAGE 29):

What is the name of Emily Bishop's husband who dies in an armed robbery gone wrong?

    a. Henry (Harry)

    b. Ernest (Ernie)

    c. Robert (Bobby)

THE COUPLE'S SCANDAL: DEIRDRE AND MIKE'S AFFAIR (PAGE 31):

What is Mike Baldwin's job at the time of his affair with Deirdre (and for most of his time on _Coronation Street_)?

    a. Factory boss

    b. Postal worker

    c. Fitness coach

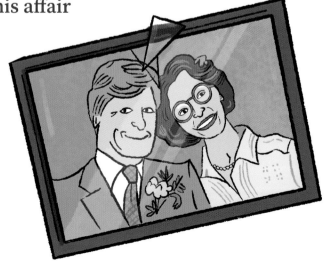

Classic couple one: Vera and Jack (page 33):

What type of birds does Jack own? Owners of this type of bird are often called 'fanciers'!

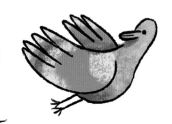

  a. Budgerigars
  b. Racing pigeons
  c. Parakeets

Classic couple two: Hilda and Stan (page 35):

What is the name of Stan and Hilda Ogden's lodger?

  a. Freddy Gates
  b. Teddy Bates
  c. Eddie Yeats

Births on The Street, Christmas 1990 (page 37):

What is the name of Gail's mum and proud grandmother of Nicky, Sarah Louise and David?

  a. Hilda
  b. Martina
  c. Audrey

SOME MORE ...

Here are some questions where the answers aren't in the book!
Each question is worth one point (except the last, which is worth five).
There is a total of sixteen points to get. The answers are on pages 71-73.

1. Which character, played by Bryan Mosley, first appears in *Coronation Street* in 1961. He becomes Mayor of Weatherfield and the owner of the minimarket?

   a. Ralf Norberts
   b. Alf Roberts
   c. Rob Alfreds

2. What is the name of Brian Tilsley's mother, played by Lynne Perrie? She is left a widow after Brian's dad, Bert, dies and would later marry cabbie, Don Brennan.

   a. Ivy
   b. Martha
   c. Ena

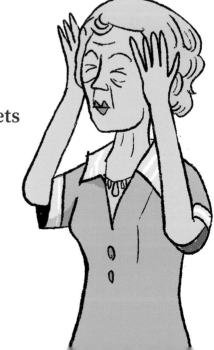

3. Who jilts her groom, Leonard Swindley, when she gets cold feet on their wedding day in 1964?

   a. Emily Nugent
   b. Concepta Hewitt
   c. Florrie Lindley

4. Who is the first husband of Deirdre (née Hunt and later Barlow), the biological father of Tracy and business partner of Len Fairclough?

a. Bobby Ewing
b. Ray Langton
c. Blake Carrington

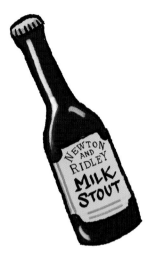

5. Which character, played by Sue Nicholls, was once the Lady Mayoress of Weatherfield?

a. Audrey (née Potter)
b. Sally (née Seddon)
c. Phyllis (née Grimes)

6. What tragically kills Ken's mother, Ida Barlow, in 1961?

a. A previously unexploded World War II bomb
b. Her neighbour's dog
c. A bus

7. Emily Bishop's lodger, who would later live with Jack and Vera Duckworth, has the character name of Norman Watts and is played by Kevin Kennedy. For somebody with such straight hair, he's given an amusing nickname. What is it?

a. Perm Boy
b. Ringlets
c. Curly

8. Is this statement true or false? In the 1970s, as well as running The Kabin, Rita Fairclough (née Littlewood) was also a nightclub singer.

a. True
b. False

9. Valerie marries Ken Barlow in 1962 after she comes to The Street to live with her Uncle Albert. What is Albert's surname, which is also Valerie's maiden name?

   a. Trotter
   b. Einstein
   c. Tatlock

10. Ena Sharples was played by which actress?

    a. Violet Carson
    b. Rose Darson
    c. Daisy Garson

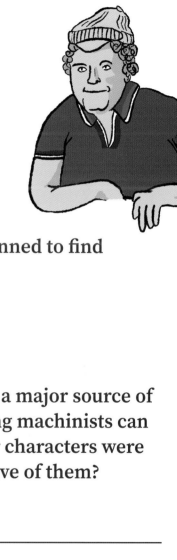

11. What unusual creatures were Annie and Jack Walker stunned to find sploshing around in their bath in 1962?

    a. Elephants
    b. Tigers
    c. Sea lions

12. Baldwin's Casuals is Mike Baldwin's clothing factory and a major source of employment in Weatherfield. In many a scene, the sewing machinists can be seen chatting away. Other than Mike, thirteen regular characters were employed there between 1976 and 1989. Can you name five of them? There's one point for each character.

_____ _____

_____ _____

_____

DID WE KNOW?

Some facts about the story of *Coronation Street* that aren't so well known.

? *Did we know* that the programme's original title was *Florizel Street*? But a tea lady at Granada Television suggested that 'Florizel' sounded like a disinfectant! From then it became known as the now-familiar *Coronation Street*.

? *Did we know* that *Coronation Street* was broadcast in black and white from the first episode in 1960? We saw the residents of Weatherfield in colour on our screens for the first time in 1969.

? *Did we know* that the first baby born on The Street was Paul Cheveski in June 1961? Paul was the son of Linda and Ivan Cheveski, and the grandson of none other than Elsie Tanner, who was just thirty-eight years old at the time!

? *Did we know* that The Rovers Return's first barmaid in 1960 was Irishwoman Concepta Riley? The pub's longest-serving barmaid was Betty Turpin (later Williams), who could be found behind the pumps for forty-three years!

? *Did we know* that two future Oscar winners have appeared on *Coronation Street*? Sir Ben Kingsley played Ron Jenkins, who took a shine to Irma Barlow in the mid-60s. Sir Ben won the Best Actor Oscar for *Gandhi* in 1983! Brenda Fricker won Best Supporting Actress in 1990 for *My Left Foot*. Back in 1977, Fricker played Staff Nurse Maloney who worked on the maternity ward when Deirdre gave birth to Tracy.

? Did we know that *Corrie* character Elaine Perkins made eight appearances as Wilfred Perkins' daughter and Ken Barlow's lover? Joanna Lumley played Elaine and her television career blossomed in such shows as *The New Avengers*, *Sapphire and Steel* and *Absolutely Fabulous*!

? *Did we know* that other famous performers who have appeared on the programme include writer and comedian, Dame Maureen Lipman, Shakespeare actor and star of *Lord of the Rings*, Sir Ian McKellen, funnyman Sir Norman Wisdom, Dame Patricia Routledge of *Keeping Up Appearances*, Bond Girl Honor Blackman and *The Professionals'* Martin Shaw?

? *Did we know* that Colin Lomax, Ena Sharples' grandson, made one appearance in 1961, played by Davy Jones? Jones went on to achieve fame in music and television with US pop group, The Monkees! The Monkees' hits included 'Daydream Believer' and 'Last Train to Clarksville'.

Did we know that other popstars have appeared in the soap? Peter Noone portrayed Len Fairclough's son, Stanley, before he was in Herman's Hermits. Others include West End star Michael Ball, The Spice Girls' Melanie B, Slade frontman Noddy Holder and rock group Status Quo.

Did we know that future acclaimed movie and television directors spent their early careers on The Street? Mike Newell would go on to direct *Four Weddings and a Funeral*, James Bond film *The World is Not Enough* had Michael Apted calling the shots, and Charles Sturridge was the director of *Brideshead Revisited*.

Did we know that the original houses on the *Coronation Street* set were built inside Granada's studios to a three-quarter size scale with cobbles painted on the studio floor? The set was rebuilt outside in 1968, before moving again in 1982. Its final rebuild was unveiled to the public at its current location of Salford Quays in 2013.

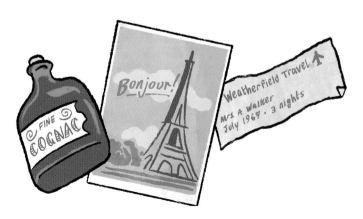

? *Did we know* that Queen Elizabeth II visited the set of *Coronation Street* in 1982 and 2021? There was also another significant royal visit to Weatherfield! Prince Charles, now King Charles III, actually appeared in a special episode to mark the show's fortieth anniversary in 2000!

? *Did we know* that Hilda Ogden was not only famed for her screechy singing, but also her English language errors? These included referring to her mountain landscape wall mural as a 'Muriel', saying Elsie Tanner's new racy bathroom was 'phonographic' and being concerned that Eddie and Stan's home brew venture would create trouble with 'customs and exercise'!

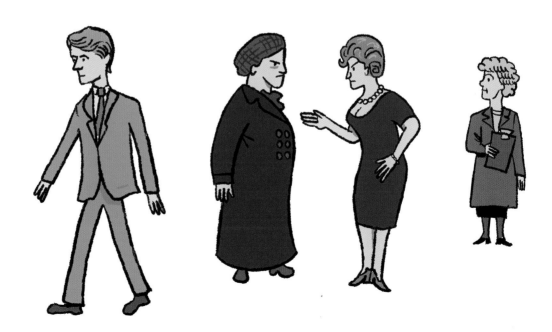

LET'S CHAT

Here are some conversation topics for you to talk about – or even just think about. There's also some space to write notes if needed.

Which character or characters did you enjoy watching on *Coronation Street*? What is it about them that you liked? Was there anything that you disliked about them – if so, what? There are some reminders later in the book (pages 55 to 68), which may prompt your thoughts.

Which storylines in *Coronation Street* stood out for you? Who was involved? Was the story tragic, or funny, or a bit of both? What was it about the storyline which made it stand out? There are some reminders on pages 58 to 63, which may prompt your thoughts.

Who did you watch *Coronation Street* with and who did you talk to about it – if anyone? How did the lives and personalities of the characters reflect your life and the lives of people around you?

What other major events can you think of from the 1960s, 1970s and 1980s? Perhaps from the music world, television, the news or even your own, or your family and friends', lives from that time?

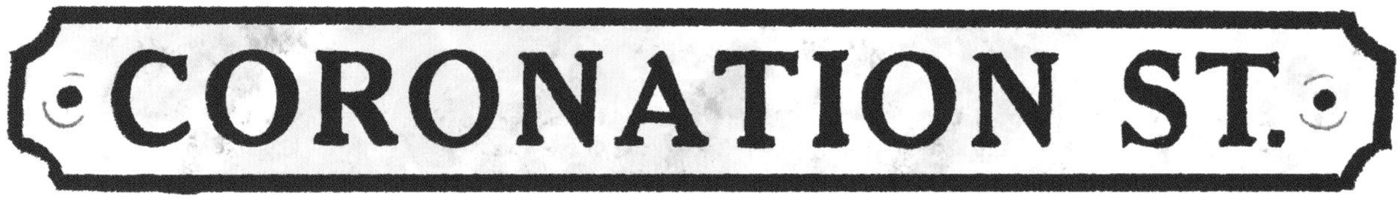
CORONATION ST.

EXPLORING WEATHERFIELD FURTHER

1983

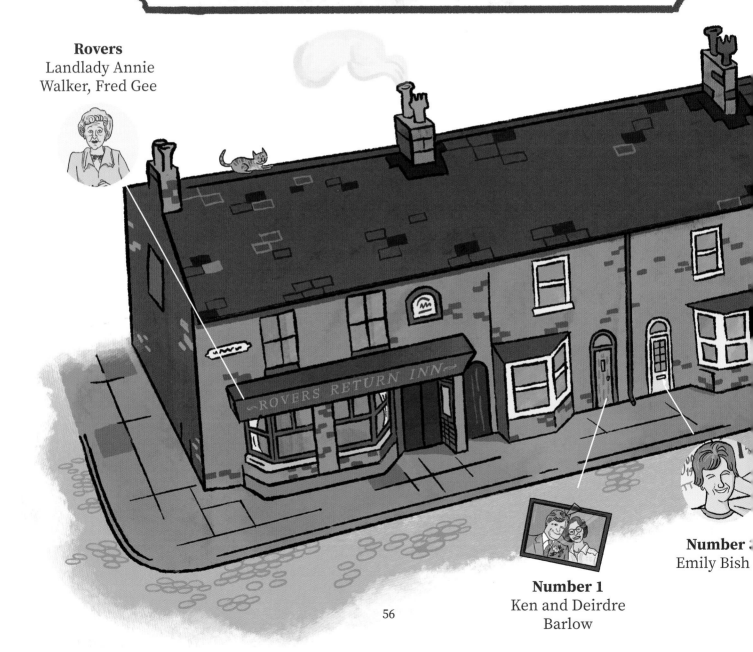

CORONATION ST.

Rovers
Landlady Annie
Walker, Fred Gee

Number 1
Ken and Deirdre
Barlow

Number 3
Emily Bish

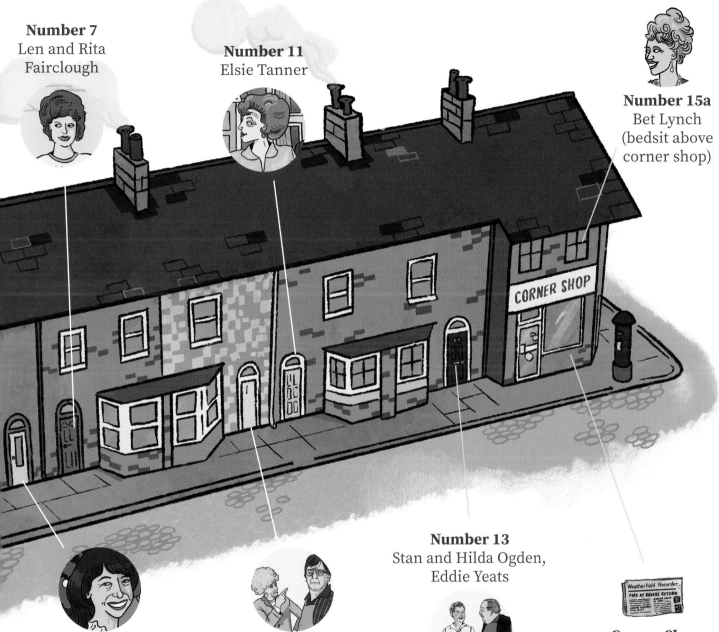

Number 7
Len and Rita Fairclough

Number 11
Elsie Tanner

Number 15a
Bet Lynch
(bedsit above corner shop)

CORNER SHOP

Number 13
Stan and Hilda Ogden, Eddie Yeats

Number 5
Ivy, Bert, Brian, Gail and Nicky Tilsley

Number 9
Jack, Vera and Terry Duckworth

Corner Shop
Alf Roberts
(downstairs living quarters)

THE *CORONATION STREET* STORY THROUGH THE DECADES: 1960s

Plot summaries from *Coronation Street* that grabbed viewers' attention in the 1960s.

Ida Barlow's death, 1961

Ken is due to move to Surrey for work, but tragedy strikes when his mother, Ida, is killed by a bus. In order to support his father, Frank, Ken makes the decision to stay in Weatherfield and marries Valerie Tatlock a year later. The residents rally around the Barlows, demonstrating The Street's tight-knit community spirit.

Will she? Won't she? Elsie and Len, 1963 (see page 21)

With Len Fairclough's split from wife, Nellie, he finds compassion and companionship in old friend, Elsie Tanner. With his divorce due to come through, Len proposes marriage. Elsie seriously considers the idea with her son, Dennis, and even Ena, encouraging her to accept. However, Elsie puts their friendship first and rejects Len's proposal.

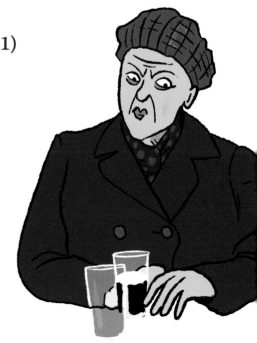

The death of Vera Lomax, 1967

Vera is the daughter of Ena Sharples, but the pair never saw eye to eye and were estranged. When Vera returns to The Street claiming to be unwell, Ena doesn't believe her. But the doctor confirms that her daughter has a terminal brain tumour. Ena can't bring herself to tell her daughter how ill she is and she's distraught after nursing Vera through her death.

Valerie Barlow held captive, 1968

An escaped prisoner, Frank Riley, takes Valerie Barlow hostage in her own home. Fearing for her twin children, Peter and Susan, Valerie bangs on the waterpipes to alert her neighbour, Ena Sharples. The police are searching for Riley and close in on their target. Despite being threatened with an iron bar, the police rescue Valerie, but she's traumatised by the events.

The Lake District coach crash, 1969

Emily Nugent (later Emily Bishop) organises a coach trip to the Lake District. But the driver, Reg Ellis, has taken a coach with faulty steering … the police are alerted, creating a race against time! The police catch up with the vehicle on the journey back to Weatherfield, but it's too late! The coach crashes and the passengers are taken to hospital. Sadly, Reg dies from his injuries.

THE *CORONATION STREET* STORY THROUGH THE DECADES: 1970S

Plot summaries from *Coronation Street* that grabbed viewers' attention in the 1970s.

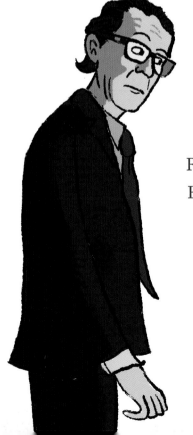

Valerie Barlow dies, 1971 (see page 29)

Ken and Valerie Barlow are moving to Jamaica, so Annie Walker throws a party for them at The Rovers. Ken's already there and Valerie rushes to get ready. Wet from her bath and struggling to fix the plug on her hairdryer, she plugs it in – still faulty – and is immediately electrocuted before their maisonette burns down!

The Kabin opens, 1973

Rita Littlewood's singing career is moving in the wrong direction. Her future husband, Len Fairclough, opens a newsagent and café called The Kabin and appoints Rita as manager. She recruits Mavis Riley as her assistant, beginning the pair's double act behind The Kabin's counter!

Hilda and Stan's second honeymoon, 1977

Hilda and Stan have a day and a night in a luxury hotel as a second honeymoon. Hilda enjoys the room service, especially the champagne. She persuades Stan to kiss her and he asks, 'What's that lipstick taste of?' To which Hilda replies, 'Woman, Stanley, woman!' Hilda sings herself to sleep, content, for once, to experience how the other half live.

Ernest Bishop is shot, 1978 (see page 29)

Ernest has a job as a wage clerk at Baldwin's Casuals and it's bonus day. Little does he realise that tragedy would strike when a robbery goes wrong! Tommo and Dave follow Ernie back to the factory, armed with a shotgun. When Mike Baldwin walks in, Tommo accidentally fires the shotgun at Ernest. He dies in hospital, leaving Emily Bishop a widow.

Lorry crashes into The Rovers, 1979 (see page 25)

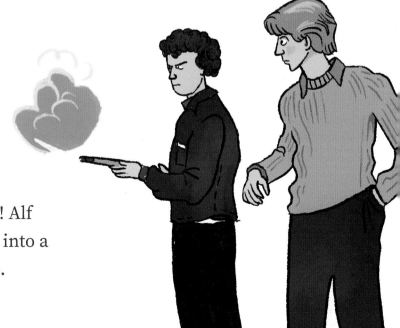

A lorry crashes into The Rovers Return, shedding its load and killing its driver. Deirdre thinks that her daughter, Tracy, is trapped in the rubble and is convinced she's dead. Fire crews do not find her in the wreckage, so Tracy is fortunately safe! Alf Roberts suffers a fractured skull and falls into a coma, from which he eventually recovers.

THE CORONATION STREET STORY THROUGH THE DECADES: 1980S

Plot summaries from *Coronation Street* that grabbed viewers' attention in the 1980s.

Emily falls for a bigamist, 1980

Emily finds love again when she marries pet shop owner, Arnold Swain, who claims to be a widower. When an insurance agent asks for Mrs Swain's signature, Emily discovers that Arnold already has a wife living in Sussex! He leaves the scene when Emily calls the police.

Mr and Mrs at The Rovers, 1981

It's a *Mr and Mrs* night at The Rovers, as Bet and Rita compere the competition to discover who knows their partner the best. Hilda is determined to win but, naturally, it all goes wrong. Stan says Hilda's perfume smells like fish and chips! Gail and Brian Tilsley are crowned champions, whilst Vera and Jack Duckworth finish last after some risqué jokes from Jack!

Vera catches Jack out, 1983

Wannabe playboy, Jack Duckworth, has joined a dating agency. His wife, Vera, finds out and hatches a plan with the help of Bet Lynch. Jack – masquerading as 'Vince St Clair' – arranges to meet mystery redhead, 'Carole Munro', in a crowded Rovers. Carole turns to reveal that she is, in fact, Vera, humiliating Jack in front of everybody!

Stan Ogden's funeral, 1984

After her husband, Stan, dies of a heart attack, Hilda Ogden busies herself preparing for his funeral at their home. The neighbourhood pulls round to support her, making sure that everything is taken care of. She hosts with care until the last guest leaves. Once the house is empty, she opens Stan's returned belongings from the hospital and sobs uncontrollably at the sight of his spectacles.

Who's the father of Gail's baby? 1986

Following an affair with husband Brian's cousin, Ian Latimer, Gail Tilsley falls pregnant. Brian finds out about her affair, and she cannot be certain if the baby is his. Brian announces this news to the entire Rovers! When baby Sarah Louise is born, a blood test confirms that she's indeed a Tilsley. Despite all this, Gail and Brian eventually work through it.

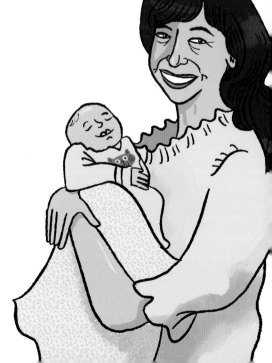

Quick Facts: 1960-1990

Here's some information about the years featured in *Classic Coronation Street*. How many of us were watching the show, the top-selling single and the Best Picture Oscar winner for each year.

	CORONATION STREET Number of viewers for most watched show[1]	POPULAR MUSIC Top-selling single[2]	MOVIES Best Picture Oscar winner[3]
1960	8.5 million (30th December)	'It's Now or Never' by Elvis Presley	*Ben Hur*
1961	16.5 million (29th November)	'Wooden Heart' by Elvis Presley	*The Apartment*
1962	19.5 million (8th October)	'I Remember You' by Frank Ifield	*West Side Story*
1963	20.2 million (18th November)	'She Loves You' by The Beatles	*Lawrence of Arabia*
1964	21.4 million (12th October)	'Can't Buy Me Love' by The Beatles	*Tom Jones*
1965	21.2 million (20th January)	'Tears' by Ken Dodd	*My Fair Lady*
1966	19.9 million (26th October)	'Green, Green Grass of Home' by Tom Jones	*The Sound of Music*
1967	20.8 million (4th September)	'Release Me' by Engelbert Humperdinck	*A Man for All Seasons*
1968	19.1 million (8th January)	'Hey Jude' by The Beatles	*In the Heat of the Night*

	CORONATION STREET Number of viewers for most watched show[1]	POPULAR MUSIC Top-selling single[2]	MOVIES Best Picture Oscar winner[3]
1969	18.4 million (26th February)	'Sugar, Sugar' by The Archies	*Oliver!*
1970	18.5 million (18th February)	'The Wonder of You' by Elvis Presley	*Midnight Cowboy*
1971	19.0 million (8th February)	'My Sweet Lord' by George Harrison	*Patton*
1972	18.3 million (5th April)	'Amazing Grace' by Royal Scots Dragoon Guards	*The French Connection*
1973	18.2 million (17th October)	'Tie a Yellow Ribbon Round the Ole Oak Tree' by Dawn featuring Tony Orlando	*The Godfather*
1974	18.3 million (20th March)	'Tiger Feet' by Mud	*The Sting*
1975	19.3 million (29th January)	'Bye Bye Baby' by The Bay City Rollers	*The Godfather Part II*
1976	19.4 million (7th April)	'Save Your Kisses for Me' by Brotherhood of Man	*One Flew Over the Cuckoo's Nest*
1977	20.9 million (20th April)	'Mull of Kintyre' by Wings	*Rocky*
1978	20.4 million (20th December)	'Rivers of Babylon' / 'Brown Girl in the Ring' by Boney M	*Annie Hall*
1979	19.5 million (14th March)	'Bright Eyes' by Art Garfunkel	*The Deer Hunter*

	CORONATION STREET Number of viewers for most watched show[1]	POPULAR MUSIC Top-selling single[2]	MOVIES Best Picture Oscar winner[3]
1980	19.0 million (3rd December)	'Don't Stand So Close to Me' by The Police	*Kramer vs. Kramer*
1981	20.8 million (18th February)	'Tainted Love' by Soft Cell	*Ordinary People*
1982	19.0 million (6th January)	'Come on Eileen' by Dexy's Midnight Runners	*Chariots of Fire*
1983	18.5 million (23rd February)	'Karma Chameleon' by Culture Club	*Gandhi*
1984	20.5 million (14th November)	'Do They Know It's Christmas?' by Band Aid	*Terms of Endearment*
1985	21.4 million (2nd January)	'The Power of Love' by Jennifer Rush	*Amadeus*
1986	19.3 million (24th February)	'Don't Leave Me This Way' by The Communards	*Out of Africa*
1987	19.8 million (14th January)	'Never Gonna Give You Up' by Rick Astley	*Platoon*
1988	18.1 million (4th January)	'Mistletoe and Wine' by Cliff Richard	*The Last Emperor*
1989	19.0 million (20th March)	'Ride on Time' by Black Box	*Rain Man*
1990	19.2 million (1st January)	'Unchained Melody' by The Righteous Brothers	*Driving Miss Daisy*

1. According to Corriepedia, *Coronation Street* Wiki (coronationstreet.fandom.com) – does not include repeats.
2. According to The Official UK Charts Company.
3. According to imdb.com – the Academy Award for Best Picture is awarded early in the year after the film's release (so the 1960 winner was released in 1959).

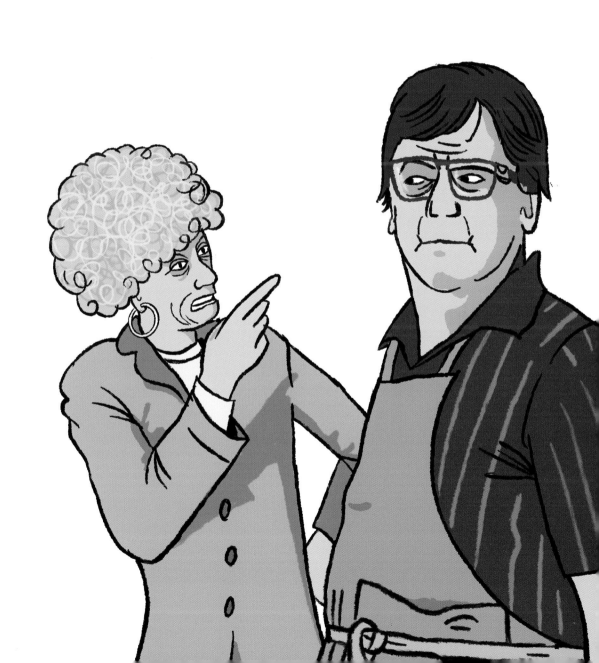

GO FURTHER INTO THE WORLD OF CORONATION STREET!

ITV X:
Keep up to date with those Weatherfield folk (and the occasional classic episode!): Just scan the QR code or visit **bit.ly/3Ndn64n**

Corriepedia:
Search for your favourite characters or plotlines at this site for true fans and the source for some of the information in this book: Just scan the QR code or visit **bit.ly/4eWBY2V**

Spotify:
If you have a Spotify account, why not download the playlist of all the songs mentioned in this book, as well as the *Coronation Street* theme? Just scan the QR code or visit **spoti.fi/40d9g9Z**

The *Coronation Street* Experience:
For those able to make the journey, this trip to Trafford Park, Manchester will mean experiencing the magic of Weatherfield up close! Just scan the QR code or visit **bit.ly/47XvYoc**

All links are correct at the time of going to print.

Just for fun – it's quiz time
Answers

The first episode (page 11):
a. Weatherfield

The Rovers Return regulars (page 13):
c. Martha

Legendary landlady one: Annie Walker (page 15):
a. Lucille

The classic Rovers bar staff line-up (page 17):
c. Lancashire hotpot

Legendary landlady two: Bet Lynch (page 19):
b. Alec Gilroy

The tough lass: Elsie Tanner (page 21):
a. True

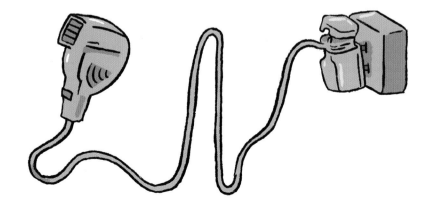

The ladies of *Coronation Street*: 1974's trip to Majorca (page 23):

c. Mavis

Disasters on The Street (page 25):

a. Tracy

The disastrous relationship of Alan Bradley and Rita Fairclough (page 27):

a. Blackpool

Deaths on The Street (page 29):

b. Ernest (Ernie)

The couple's scandal: Deirdre and Mike's affair (page 31):

a. Factory boss

Classic couple one: Vera and Jack (page 33):

b. Racing pigeons

Classic couple two: Hilda and Stan (page 35):

c. Eddie Yeats

Births on The Street, Christmas 1990 (page 37):

c. Audrey

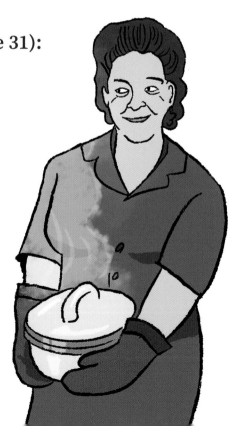

Some more ...
Answers

1. Which character, played by Bryan Mosley, first appears in *Coronation Street* in 1961?

   b. Alf Roberts

2. What is the name of Brian Tilsley's mother, played by Lynne Perrie?

   a. Ivy

3. Who jilts her groom, Leonard Swindley, when she gets cold feet on their wedding day in 1964?

   a. Emily Nugent

4. Who is the first husband of Deirdre (née Hunt and later Barlow), the biological father of Tracy and business partner of Len Fairclough?

   b. Ray Langton

5. Which character, played by Sue Nicholls, was once the Lady Mayoress of Weatherfield?

   a. Audrey (née Potter)

6. What tragically kills Ken's mother, Ida Barlow, in 1961?

   c. A bus

7. Emily Bishop's lodger, who would later live with Jack and Vera Duckworth, has the character name of Norman Watts and is played by Kevin Kennedy. For somebody with such straight hair, he's given an amusing nickname. What is it?

   c. Curly

8. Is this statement true or false? In the 1970s, as well as running The Kabin, Rita Fairclough (née Littlewood) was also a nightclub singer.

   a. True

9. Valerie marries Ken Barlow in 1962 after she came to The Street to live with her Uncle Albert. What is Albert's surname, which is also Valerie's maiden name?

   c. Tatlock

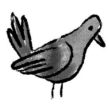
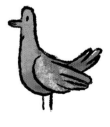

10. Ena Sharples was played by which actress?

    a. Violet Carson

11. What unusual creatures were Annie and Jack Walker stunned to find sploshing around in their bath in 1962?

    c. Sea lions

12. Baldwin's Casuals is Mike Baldwin's clothing factory and a major source of employment in Weatherfield. In many a scene, the sewing machinists can be seen chatting away. Other than Mike, thirteen regular characters were employed there between 1976 and 1989. Can you name five of them? There's one point for each character.

Elsie Tanner
Ernest Bishop
Emily Bishop
Fred Gee
George Wardle
Hilda Ogden
Ida Clough
Ivy Tilsley
Shirley Armitage
Steve Fisher
Suzie Birchall
Terry Duckworth
Vera Duckworth.

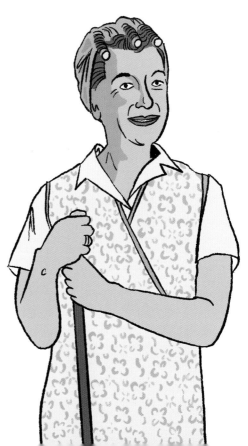

ALL ABOUT ME

a picture of me

In this section, you can share some things that are personal to you. It's great to do these things in twos if there's someone else who knows you well!

Name:
....

Date of birth:
....

Birthplace:
....

People who are important to me:
....

....

My favourite films:
....

....

My favourite music:
....

....

My favourite book:

....

....

My favourite food:

....

....

My favourite drink:

....

....

My favourite places:

....

....

Things that make me laugh:

....

....

Things that make me cry:

....

....

Supporters' guide

This section is for the loved ones or carers of the reader, who can enjoy the book too! Here are some useful hints and tips to make sure everyone gets the most out of their Cognitive Book.

Scan here for the audio!

1

Follow the instructions to download the free audio at:
cognitivebooks.co.uk/download

2

The audio really helps support the enjoyment of a Cognitive Book! Encourage the reader – if they are able – to read along while listening.

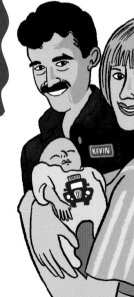

3 Don't leave this book in amongst other books – like on a bookshelf or in a pile by the bedside.

● ●

Always leave the book somewhere it's frequently to hand and easy to access – the armrest of the sofa or a table near where the reader regularly sits, or the bedside table if they like to read at night, for example.

4

For those finding reading more difficult these days, it might be better to stick to the left-hand page of each spread to enjoy the simpler text and vibrant illustrations.

Many readers will be able to explore a Cognitive Book largely on their own – the full text on the right-hand page of each spread will often be accessible to them.

5  **6**

7

Pages 39 to 53 contain exercises you can work on together. Try to support the reader in answering the quiz questions (pages 40-47) and give prompts for the 'Let's chat' questions (page 52). You can also explore Weatherfield further with them (pages 55-68)!

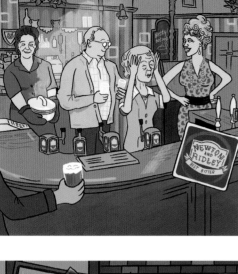

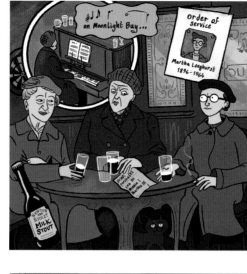

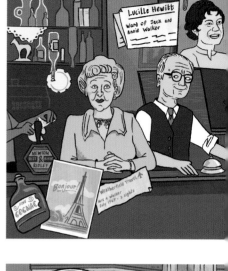

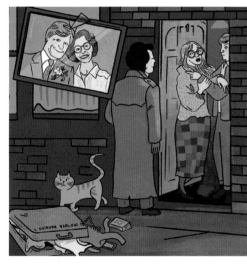

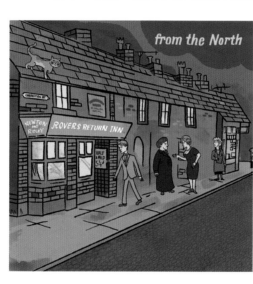

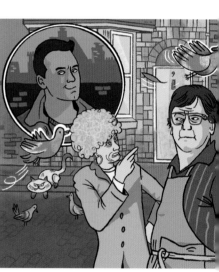

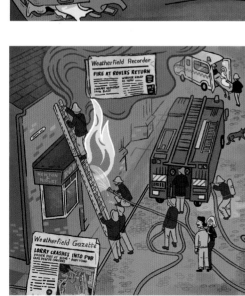

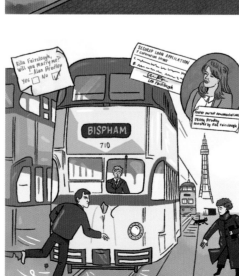

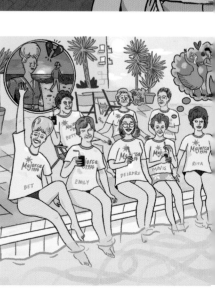

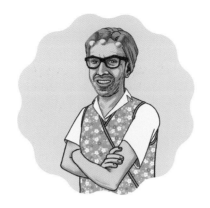

Cognitive Books are enjoyed by everyone.

I started writing these books for my dad, Brian. I wanted to create something he'd enjoy today but, equally, something I know he'd have taken pleasure in reading twenty years ago. They're designed to be fun, stimulating and something that can be enjoyed alone, or – if preferred – with a supporter, such as a loved one or a carer.

After testing the books with Alzheimer's Society, we realised just how suitable they are for people with dementia or other cognitive difficulties. Brian, who happens to be living with dementia, loves *looking back at … The Beatles* and *looking back at … The 1966 World Cup.* We hope you enjoy their follow-up, *looking back at … Classic Coronation Street,* as much as he enjoys his Cognitive Books!

Sign up to our mailing list at **cognitivebooks.co.uk** to discover future titles.

Happy reading!

Matt

Matt Singleton
Author and director of Cognitive Books
cognitivebooks.co.uk

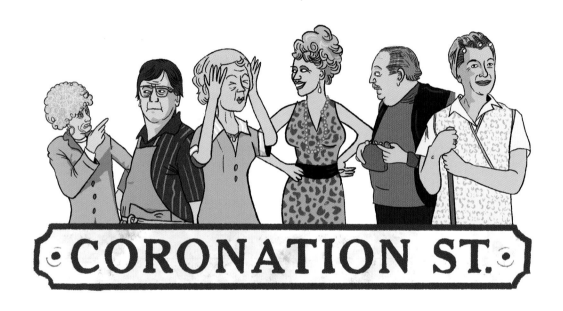

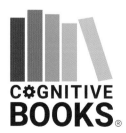